Gluten Free Diet

The Secret to a Healthy Gut

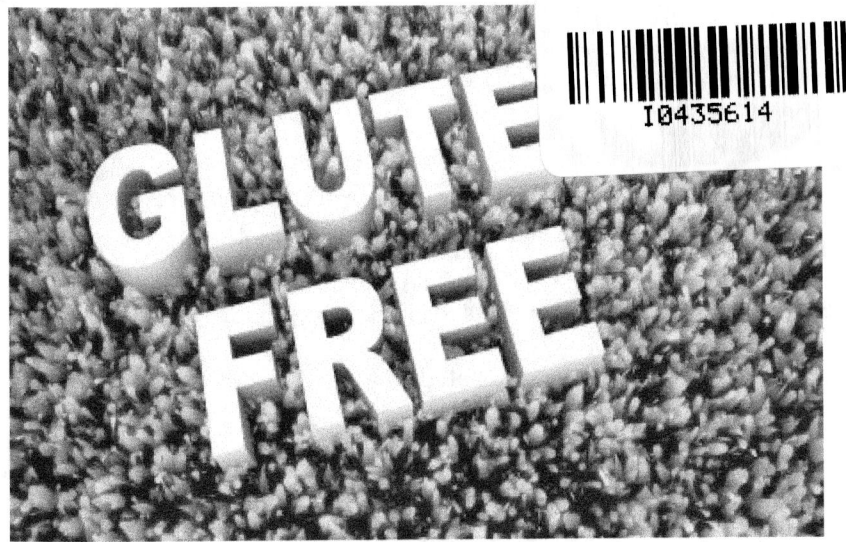

Health Learning Series

M. Usman

Mendon Cottage Books

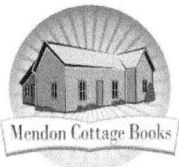

JD-Biz Publishing

Disclaimer

The information is this book is provided for informational purposes only. It is not intended to be used and medical advice or a substitute for proper medical treatment by a qualified health care provider. The information is believed to be accurate as presented based on research by the author.

The contents have not been evaluated by the U.S. Food and Drug Administration or any other Government or Health Organization and the contents in this book are not to be used to treat cure or prevent disease.

The author or publisher is not responsible for the use or safety of any diet, procedure, or treatment mentioned in this book. The author or publisher is not responsible for errors or omissions that may exist.

Warning

The Book is for informational purposes only and before taking on any diet, treatment or medical procedure, it is recommended to consult with your primary health care provider.

Our books are available at

1. Amazon.com
2. Barnes and Noble
3. Itunes
4. Kobo
5. Smashwords
6. Google Play Books

Table of Contents

Prelude

The Celiac disease is a disorder that is not unheard of. People who suffer from this disorder are prone to stomach damage if they consume foods containing gluten. A gluten-free diet specifically targets these people and is thus a diet that excludes foods containing gluten.

When consumed, gluten causes inflammation in the small intestine that leads to other signs and symptoms. In order to prevent and bring these signs under check, gluten must be avoided. Any person, unless of course an experienced medical practitioner, cannot build his/her own diet out of scratch, even though the diet's name is pretty much self-explanatory.

This is where this book comes in; it relieves you of any doubt about the causes of the problems the diet deals with, to its recipes, so you would have complete knowledge when you shift to the non-gluten regimen. Moreover, the diet is also applicable to people with non-celiac gluten sensitivity which will be explained later. Note that people with non-celiac gluten sensitivity may or may not benefit from a gluten-free diet, but for sufferers of celiac disease, a gluten-free meal plan is a necessity rather than a suggestion.

Switching to the diet can itself be a big step as it will pretty much involve you to substitute each gluten component of your diet with something new. But with courage, faith, and guidance in the right direction, it is not that difficult to accomplish this goal.

Read on and find out more!

Celiac Disease

Chapter # 1: Overview

Celiac disease affects people all round the globe. Once it was thought of as nothing but a rare childhood disorder, in other words, nothing to be worried about, but now it has grown into a full blown health problem with millions of dollars' worth of medical research being carried out on it. It is a common genetic disorder nowadays which rattles over 2 million people in the United States alone. In people who have a first degree relation with a carrier of celiac disease, it has a probability of 1/22. Also the Celiac disease is more common with people who have another genetic disorder such as Turner or Down syndrome.

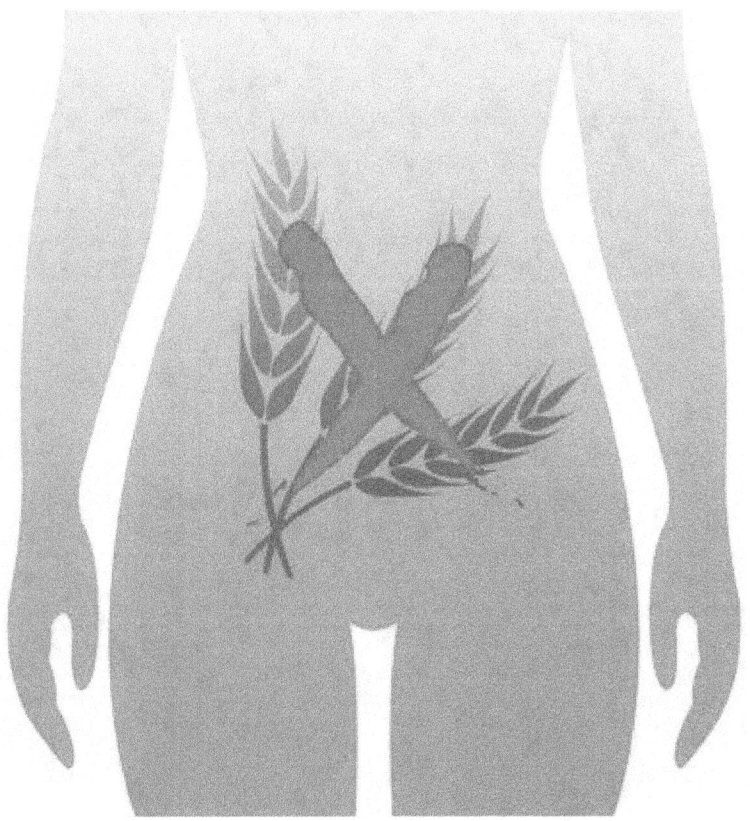

Celiac disease is a disease that targets the digestive system and damages different organs, primarily the small intestine, interfering with its natural processes like absorption of nutrients from the food. People who have this disease cannot tolerate **gluten** which is a protein found in different food items like rye, barley and wheat. Gluten is found in foods and everyday products, but is normally labeled. When people with Celiac disease consume gluten their immune system malfunctions and responds with the destruction of villi, which are the lining on the small intestine that allow nutrients to be absorbed through the walls of the intestine. Without a healthy lining a person faces malnourishment no matter how much he puts in!

Chapter # 2: Symptoms

Symptoms of the disease vary quite differently from one person to the other. These signs may develop in any part of the body ranging from intestinal organs to the skin. In young children and infants the disease takes its tolls on the digestive system; symptoms include:

- Chronic diarrhea,

- Abdominal pain and bloating,

- Constipation,

- Vomiting,

- Weight loss,

- Pale, foul-smelling stool,

These symptoms may be accompanied by irritability.

This disease can really dent a child's growth, as lack of nutrients during this period affects the child's natural development, and can cause problems in the future like dental defects, short stature, puberty problems, etc.

Adults are less likely to have these digestive issues and may suffer from:

- Anemia,

- Bone or joint pain,

- Fatigue,

- Bone loss,

- Arthritis,

- Depression,

- Seizures,

- Tingling or numbness,

- Missed menstrual periods,

- Itchy skin rash,

- Sores inside the mouth

Long term complications of the disease include osteoporosis, anemia, and miscarriage.

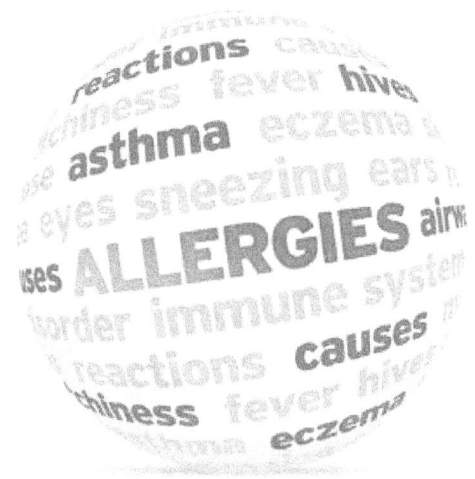

Researchers are still putting effort into the widely asked question as to why celiac disease affects different people, differently. The length of time a child is breastfed, the length of time before the child made contact with gluten, and the amount of gluten he/she eats are 3 of the most important factors that govern the behavior of the disease. Some studies have shown that when children were breastfed for a longer period of time, they were protected from celiac disease for a fairly long time compared to those who were breastfed for a shorter instance of time. Moreover, it was found that the symptoms also vary depending on a person's age and the damage that the small intestine has already suffered from. Many adults develop the disease a long time, typically a decade, before they are diagnosed. Only after the disease has ravaged the internal body organs, do they find out. The longer a person goes untreated and undiagnosed, the higher the chances of long-term problems become.

People with celiac disease also suffer from a variety of other problems that are related to the immune system. The connection between these diseases and celiac disease may or may not be genetic:

- Autoimmune thyroid disease,

- Type 1 diabetes,

- Rheumatoid arthritis,

- Addison's disease, in which the glands that produce vital hormones are damaged,

- Sjogren's disease, in which glands producing tears and saliva are injured.

Chapter # 3: Diagnostics

Just like high blood pressure is invisible to many, celiac disease can also become a silent condition and keep on affecting the body until the damage is finally visible. The disease is often consumed with many other conditions like the irritable bowel syndrome, inflammatory bowel disease, anemia, intestinal infections, and chronic fatigue. Thus, celiac disease largely goes unnoticed and the patient gets treated for the wrong ailment. As new research is telling doctors more about the disease, they are becoming increasingly aware of the disease, and the number of cases associated with misdiagnosis is dramatically decreasing.

Blood tests:

People who suffer from celiac disease have certain elements in their blood that are higher than the normal limit. Certain antibodies and other compounds that react with the body's own tissues are present in much higher amounts which leads to the denting of the body's internal structure. To diagnose celiac disease doctors test the blood for high levels of substances, namely:

    i.   anti-tissue transglutaminase antibodies (tTGA),

    ii.   anti-endomysium antibodies (EMA)

If test results turn out negative, but celiac disease still maintains its presence, then additional tests may be required. But, before one administers such a test, he/she must eat a diet filled with gluten like pastas, bread or cereal. If a person stops eating gluten for a considerable amount of time and then goes for a test, the result would logically be negative!

Intestinal Biopsy:

If blood tests and symptoms, both suggest the presence of celiac disease, the doctors perform a biopsy of the small intestine so that the earlier diagnostics can be made crystal clear. During the biopsy, the doctor checks the tissue of the small intestine for damage done to the villi. In order to obtain the tissue, the doctor carries a tedious procedure which involves placing an endoscope through the patient's mouth into his/her stomach.

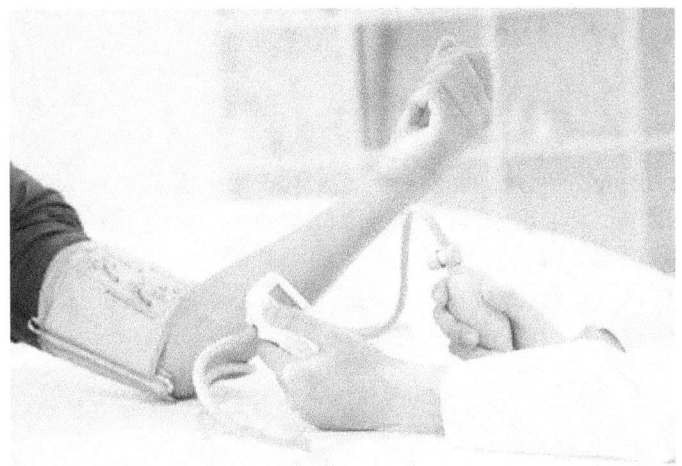

Screening:

Celiac disease is also screened in many countries, which means checking for the presence of auto-antibodies in one's blood. Americans routinely go through this process of screening, but as celiac disease may be contracted via genes, all family members of a person carrying the disease must go through this process.

The Case of Dermatitis Herpetiformis:

Dermatitis Herpetiformis or DH is an extremely itchy and blistering skin rash that affects 15 – 25 % of the people that suffer from the celiac disease. The rash occurs on parts of body like knees, buttocks, and elbows. Furthermore, most people who suffer from DH don't have any digestive symptoms associated with celiac disease. DH is diagnosed via various blood tests and a biopsy of the skin. If the antibody tests turns out positive while the skin biopsy also supports this statement, then there is no further need of an intestinal biopsy. Both the intestinal disease and the skin disease have a collective response to gluten and the skin rash symptoms come back as soon as contact with gluten is made. Moreover, DH is not treated by anti-biotics therefore the person has to avoid gluten food at all times.

Gluten-Free Diet

Chapter # 1: Intro

If you are diagnosed with Celiac disease, your health care provider will recommend you to a dietitian to help you shift to a gluten-free diet. A dietitian will help you read the labels of food items and help you identify foods that contain gluten; this will help you make informed decisions when buying groceries at the supermarket.

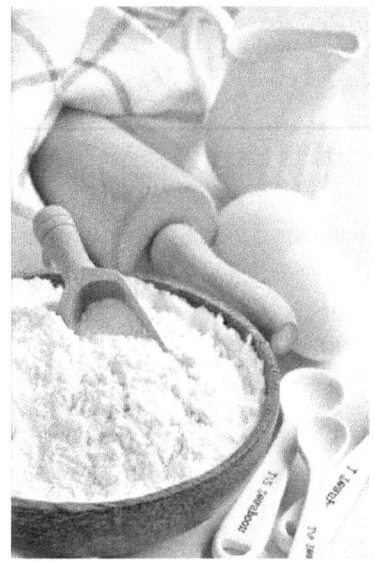

For most people, shifting over to a gluten-free diet plan would mean relief from signs and symptoms associated with the celiac disease. Marked progress can be seen within days of the shift over; the small intestine takes 3 – 6 months, depending on the damage done, to heal in the case of children, but take several years in case of an adult. A healed small intestine means villi is now performing its true function, i.e. absorbing nutrients from the food, and transferring them into the blood stream.

To stay well, sufferers of the celiac disease must avoid gluten as much as possible for the remainder of their life. Eating even a small amount of it can damage the intestinal lining and once again make life miserable. The damage can occur to anyone with the disease, even to those with the slightest symptoms. Depending on the person's age, some problems may not improve like dental and stature effects.

The most common reason, if you are still undergoing a poor response to gluten free food, is because small amounts of it are still going in your body. Hidden sources of gluten include additives, preservatives, and stabilizers. Furthermore, many gluten-free products like corn and rice are manufactured in factories that also make wheat thus, contaminating them with gluten.

Some rare cases have still appeared in which the intestinal problems continued despite a strict check on what goes in the body. People with the underlying condition suffer from something known as refractory celiac disease, which is a case of severely damaged intestines that rarely heal. Due to this the intestines are not able to absorb enough nutrients and thus the condition persists.

Chapter # 2: Going Gluten-Free

The gluten-free diet does not mean that eating foods that have rye, barley, and wheat in them should be avoided, but it means that all the products that are made from these grains should also be avoided, irrespective of their proportion in the final food item. Despite these restrictions, people with the celiac disorder can enjoy a well-balanced diet using a variety of replacements. They may use foods like rice, potatoes, quinoa, buckwheat, amaranth, or bean flour; the options are unlimited. They may purchase gluten-free breakfast and other products from stores which are becoming more and more common with every passing quarter.

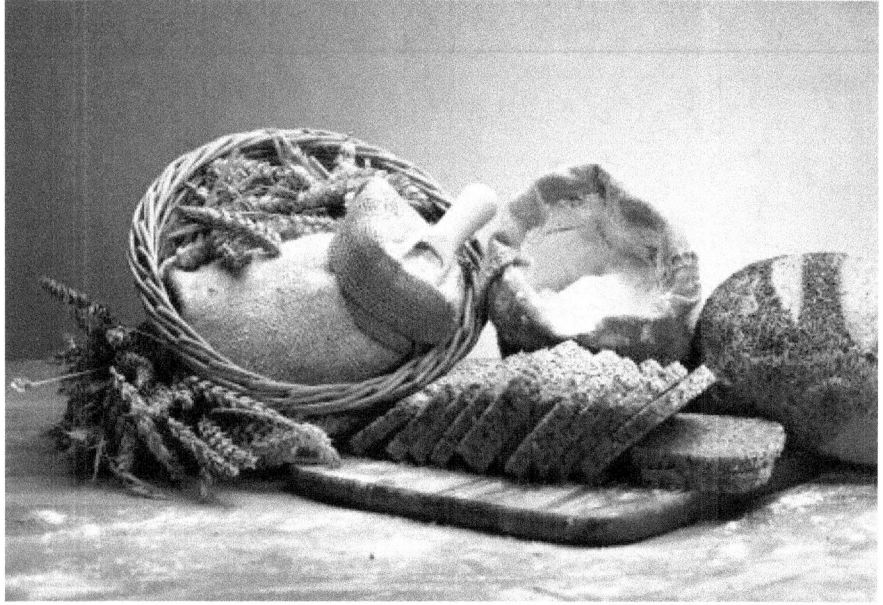

Plain meat, rice, fish, fruits, and vegetables are all food items that do not contain gluten. Therefore people with celiac disease are free to enjoy them. In the past people were advised not to eat oats, but new mounting evidence is suggesting that most people can eat small quantities of oats without making them self-prone to the disease. Oats themselves do not contain gluten, but they get processed in a factory that does, causing them to be related with gluten-containing products. New, dedicated factories are producing oats specifically for gluten-intolerant people so you can buy from these brands instead.

The gluten free diet requires a completely revamped approach to eating food. Freshly diagnosed individuals, plus their families, will find a support group quite useful to them as it will provide the emotional support needed to completely shift to a new diet plan. People with celiac disease must remain cautious at all times, e.g. school, work, etc. as the slightest mistake on their part could result in days or weeks' worth of agony. When eating outside, ask the waiter whether gluten-free food is available.

Gluten is even used in some medicines, so the doctor must be aware of this condition before prescribing you any drug! The ball is pretty much in your court now!

Chapter # 3: What to Eat?

In 2006, the US Dietetic Association updated its recommendation to the gluten-free foods list. The chart illustrating these recommendations is shown below. The list is NOT complete due to its exhaustive nature, therefore should not considered the final word. People with celiac disease should always read the ingredients in any food item before they buy it.

Allowed
Legumes, seeds, amaranth, arrowroot, cassava, buckwheat, corn, flax, Indian rice grass, Job's tears, millet, nuts, potatoes, quinoa, sago, rice, sorghum, tapioca, soy, wild rice, yucca, teff
Foods to Avoid
Wheat including emmer, spelt, kamut, einkorn, wheat bran, wheat starch, cracked wheat, wheat germ
Barley, tritacle, rye
Other Wheat Containing Products
Self-rising flour, durum flour, graham flour, bromated flour, phosphate flour, semolina, enriched flour, farina, plain flour, white flour
Processed Foods that have Gluten
French fries, gravy, imitation fish, sauces, rice mixes, bouillon cubes, candy, brown rice syrup, potato chips, hot dogs, salami, cold cuts, communion wafers, soups, soy sauce, self-basting turkey, seasoned tortilla chips

The complete list as given by Massachusetts General Hospital is as follows:

Allowed	Not Allowed
Grains & Starches	
Tapioca; soybean; arrowroot; potato	Wheat; white or whole wheat flour;

flours. Buckwheat; quinoa; amaranth; millet; teff; sourghum (Milo); flax. Rice; cream-of-rice; wild rice. Corn; unflavored popcorn; cornmeal, hominy; grits; corn starch Pure, gluten-free oats. Ready-to-eat cereal made from allowed grains; gluten-free pasta.	bromated flour; enriched flour; phosphated flour; self-rising flour; graham flour; durum flour; semolina; wheat germ; bran; bulgur (tabbouleh); kamut; wheat berries; couscous; spelt; faro; emmer; einkorn; triticale; atta; dinkel. Rye; rye flour; rye bread. Barley; barley groats; barley flakes. Oats; oat groats; oat bran; oat flour. Cereals; pasta; noodles; spaghetti; farina; cream of wheat; dumplings; bread; bakery bread; rolls; stuffing; cake; crackers; muffins; pastries; biscuits; melba toast; zwieback; rusk; matzo; waffles; pancakes; donuts; prepared mixes; pretzels.
Beverages	
Fresh brewed coffee (no grains added); teas without prohibited grains. Milk or chocolate milk with cocoa. 100% fruit juices, soda (check labels). Wine; distilled alcohols and cordials.	Instant coffee; instant tea; some herbal teas; instant cocoa with grains added. Malted milk; flavored milk with cereal fillers added; rice or soy beverages using barley enzymes. Beverages with flavorings of unknown content or those that contain cereal grains or malt; some root beers. Beer; lagers; ales.

Soups & Casseroles

Clear, home-made broth; gluten-free bouillon cubes; soups made with rice or gluten-free pasta stock; creamed soups and chowders thickened with cream, cornstarch, potato flour or other allowed special flours. Prepared gluten-free macaroni that don't contain sauces thickened with flour; gratins made with only cream (no flour or prohibited thickeners)	Bouillon-based broths; creamed soups or chowders thickened with flour; most gumbos; prepared soups with prohibited cereal grains or thickeners. Macaroni, cheese, and casseroles in a white sauce thickened with flour (using a roux or beurre manie); dishes served with gravy, béchamel, veloute, or espagnole sauces.

Fats

Butter; oils (check label for wheat germ oil or any unidentified oil source); lard; most vegetable shortenings and margarines (check labels); foods fried in uncontaminated oils that have not been breaded with prohibited flours. Pure mayonnaise (and other salad dressings that are thickened with egg, cornstarch or allowed special flours); homemade salad dressings made with distilled vinegar Cream; bacon; nuts; olives; peanut butter; avocado; sour cream and cream cheese.	Wheat germ oil; margarines and spreads made with prohibited stabilizers; Olestra; most fried and breaded foods. Low calorie mayonnaise made with prohibited cereal thickeners; commercial salad dressings that contain wheat flour; dressings made with malt vinegar; gravies; béchamel, veloute, espagnole sauces or other sauces thickened with flour (using a rouxs or beurre manie); low fat sour creams, low fat cream cheese and any other low fat products made with prohibited ingredients.

Seasonings & Sweets

Pure spices and herbs; salt;	Marinades, seasoning mixes and

monosodium glutamate (MSG). Sugar; molasses; honey; jelly; jam; corn syrup; maple syrup; imitation or pure vanilla extract. Pure cocoa; pure chocolate; coconut; marshmallows and candies made from allowed grains. Ketchup; mustard; pickles; relish; horseradish; steak sauce not prepared with prohibited ingredients; gluten-free soy sauce. Distilled rice, wine, or cider vinegar	dips, some ground spices and curry powders containing prohibited ingredients; bouillon cubes; malt flavoring; brewer's Yeast. Malt syrup; brown rice syrup; malt extract Candy and other confections which contain prohibited ingredients or are of unknown content; Soy sauce; prepared sauces and condiments containing prohibited ingredients. Malt vinegar and vinegars made with prohibited ingredients.

Dairy

Whole, low-fat, skim, fresh, dried or evaporated milk; flavored milks (check labels). Plain yogurt and kefir; flavored yogurt and kefir (check labels). All aged hard cheeses (cheddar, parmesan, Swiss, etc.); cottage cheese (check labels).	Flavored milks made with prohibited ingredients; malted milk products. Cheese food and cheese spread made with prohibited ingredients; Roquefort cheese made with bread mold.

Fruits & Vegetables

Fresh, frozen, dried, or canned (check labels).	Fruits and pie filling containing thickeners; canned products with preservatives, emulsifiers, or food starch made from prohibited grains.

Meat or Meat Substitutes	
Fresh meat; poultry; fish and shellfish; eggs. Edamame (soy beans); tofu; beans; nuts (check labels).	Most luncheon meats, sausages and hot dogs containing prohibited grains; self-basing turkeys; animal proteins marinated using prohibited ingredients; animal proteins in sauces made with prohibited grains; imitation seafood; crabstick; sushi made with crabstick (California rolls). Seitan; soy-based meats that contain plant proteins made with prohibited ingredients; bean dips made with prohibited ingredients; dry roasted nuts containing prohibited ingredients
Miscellaneous	
	Some chewing gums. Some toothpaste; mouthwash; medicines (especially imported medicines); laxatives; vitamin supplements. Some make-up (especially lipstick and balm) Communion wafers. Glue; play dough.

The National Institute of Diabetes, Digestive and Kidney Diseases is a notable institution that conducts as well as provides support to researchers on Celiac disease. Researchers are now studying for new options that could preemptively tell them whether a person has celiac disease or not.

Furthermore, several drug treatments for celiac disease are being considered and are under evaluation. A number of enzymes and other compounds are being studied to give a better overview of the disease. Participants in clinical trials are the researcher's farthest approach to better knowing about drugs that are effective against celiac disease. Therefore, until a drug is proven effective, the non-gluten diet is the only way to tackle the celiac disease.

Main Dishes

Chapter # 1: Baked Omelet Pie

Makes: 8 servings

Prep time: 20 minutes

Cooking time: 20 minutes

Ready in: 40 minutes

Ingredients:

- 1 large potato for baking

- 6 eggs

- ½ teaspoon black pepper, ground

- 1 teaspoon salt

- 2 tablespoons olive oil

- ¼ cup fresh parsley, chopped

- ¼ cup red bell pepper, chopped

- 1 chopped onion

- ¼ cup red bell pepper, chopped

- 1 sliced tomato

- ¼ cup Cheddar cheese, shredded

Directions:

Take a medium pot of salted water and bring it to a boil. Add the potato and cook until it turns tender, but still has firmness; this will take about 15 minutes. After this, drain the potatoes and let them cool before peeling and slicing them. Preheat an oven to 175 degrees Celsius. Beat the salt, pepper, parsley, and eggs together. In a cast iron skillet, heat the olive oil over medium heat. Salute the onion and peppers until they are soft, and then add in the mushrooms. When the mushrooms show signs of shrinking, add the potato and tomato slices. Pour the egg mixture in and gently start stirring the combination. On top of the eggs, sprinkle the cheese and place the skillet in a preheated oven. Then, bake the eggs until they are firm which will take about 10 – 15 minutes. Finally, allow it to cool for some time before serving.

Chapter # 2: Barbecued Beef

Makes: 12 servings

Prep time: 20 minutes

Cooking time: 10 hours

Ready in: 10 hours 20 minutes

Ingredients:

- 1 teaspoon liquid smoke flavoring,

- 1 ½ cup ketchup

- ¼ cup red wine vinegar

- ¼ cup brown sugar

- 2 tablespoons Dijon-style mustard

- 2 tablespoons Worcestershire sauce

- ½ teaspoons salt

- ¼ teaspoon black pepper

- 1 boneless chuck roast (4 pounds)

- ¼ teaspoon garlic powder

Directions:

Take a large bowl and combine the brown sugar, ketchup, red wine vinegar, Worcestershire sauce, Dijon-style mustard, and liquid smoke. Mix in the pepper, salt, and garlic powder. Place the chuck roast in a cooker (slow) and pour the ketchup mixture prepared earlier over it. Next, cover it and cook for 8 – 10 hours. Remove the chuck roast from the cooker and shred using a fork; return it to the slow cooker. Add in the meat to coat it with the sauce evenly and continue to cook for another hour.

Chapter # 3: Stuffed Peppers

Makes: 6 servings

Prep time: 20 minutes

Cooking time: 1 hour

Ready in: 1 hour 20 minutes

Ingredients:

- 1 tablespoon Worcestershire sauce

- 1 pound ground beef

- ½ cup long grain white rice, uncooked

- 1 cup water

- 6 green bell peppers

- 2 (8 ounce) tomato sauce cans

- ¼ teaspoon onion powder

- ¼ teaspoon garlic powder

- Salt & pepper

- 1 teaspoon Italian seasoning

Directions:

Preheat an oven to 175 degrees Celsius. Place the water and rice in a saucepan and let it boil. Reduce the heat when boiling begins; cover and let it cook for 20 minutes. In a skillet, cook the beef over medium heat until it turns brown on all sides. Remove and discard the seeds, tops, and membranes of the peppers. Arrange them in a baking dish with the hollowed sides pointed upwards. Slice the bottoms if necessary so that the peppers would stand in an upward direction. In a bowl, mix the cooked rice, browned beef, and the can of tomato sauce, garlic powder, Worcestershire sauce, salt, onion powder, and pepper. Spoon out an equal quantity of the mixture onto hollowed peppers. Next, mix the tomato sauce that remains plus Italian seasoning in a bowl and pour it over the stuffed peppers. Bake for an hour in the oven and baste with sauce every 15 minutes until peppers are abundantly tender.

Chapter # 4: Lamb Chops

Makes: 4 servings

Prep time: 10 minutes

Cooking time: 15 minutes

Ready in: 40 minutes

Ingredients:

- 1 tablespoon olive oil

- ¼ teaspoon dried basil

- ¾ teaspoon dried rosemary

- ¼ cup shallots, minced

- ½ teaspoon dried thyme

- 1/3 cup balsamic vinegar

- ¾ cup chicken broth

- 1 tablespoon butter

- 4 lamb chops

- Salt & pepper to taste

Directions:

In a small cup or bowl, mix the basil, rosemary, salt, pepper, and thyme. Rub this mixture over the lamb chops on both its sides and place them on a plate. Cover it and set aside for about 15 minutes so that the chops can absorb the flavors. Take a large skillet and heat the olive oil in it over medium heat. Place the lamb chops after they have attained the flavor in it and let it cook for 3 ½ minutes on each side until it is medium rare. Remove the lamb chops and keep them warm using a platter. Add shallots in the skillet and cook for another few minutes until it turns brown. Add in the vinegar, scrap any bits of lamb from the bottom, and stir in the chicken broth. Continue cooking over medium heat for 5 minutes until only half of the sauce remains. If you don't do this then the sauce will be very runny. Finally remove from the heat and add in the butter. Pour this over the lamb chops and serve.

Chapter # 5: Mexican Style Meat

Makes: 12 servings

Prep time: 30 minutes

Cooking time: 8 hours

Ready in: 8 hours 50 minutes

Ingredients:

- 1 chuck roast (4 pound)

- 1 ¼ cups green chili pepper, diced

- 1 teaspoon chili powder

- 1 teaspoon salt

- 1 teaspoon ground cayenne pepper

- 1 teaspoon ground black pepper

- 1 bottle hot pepper sauce (5 ounce)

- 2 tablespoons olive oil

- 1 teaspoon garlic powder

- 1 large onion, chopped

Directions:

Trim the chuck roast of any fat it has and season it with pepper and salt. Take a large skillet and heat the olive oil over medium heat. Place the beef in the skillet and brown it on all sides, quickly. Transfer this into a slow cooker and top it up with some chopped onion. Season it with chili powder, chili peppers, hot pepper sauce, cayenne pepper, and garlic powder. Add abundant amount of water until 1/3 of the roast is covered. Cover and cook the roast for at least 6 hours, checking again and again to make sure that there is some liquid still left at the bottom of the cooker. Reduce the heat from high to low after 6 hours and continue to cook for 2 – 4 more hours or of course, until the meet turns extremely tender and literally falls apart. Transfer this roast onto a bowl and shred it to pieces using forks. If desired, reserve two cups of the cooking liquid and serve in burritos or tacos.

Desserts

Chapter # 1: Zucchini Bread

Makes: 1 loaf

Prep time: 15 minutes

Cooking time: 1 hour

Ready in: 1 hour 15 minutes

Ingredients:

- 1 cup zucchini, diced
- 1 teaspoon baking powder
- 2 eggs
- 1 teaspoon cinnamon, ground
- ½ cup canola oil
- ¾ teaspoon baking soda
- 1 teaspoon gluten-free vanilla
- ½ teaspoon xanthan gum
- ½ teaspoon salt
- 1 cup white sugar
- ½ cup sweet rice flour
- ½ cup white rice flour
- ½ cup cornstarch
- 1 teaspoons lemon juice

- 2 tablespoons tapioca starch

Directions:

Preheat an oven to 165 degrees Celsius; grease a loaf pan. Combine the eggs, zucchini, vanilla extract, and oil in a blender and pulse it until the mixture gives the appearance of a milkshake. Whisk the white rice flour, sweet rice flour, sugar, tapioca, baking powder, cinnamon, cornstarch, baking soda, salt, and xanthan gum. Add the zucchini mixture into the flour one and keep on battering until it is well blended. Finally pour it into the loaf pan. Bake in the oven for about an hour or until a toothpick comes out clean when inserted into the bread. Cool the pan for a few minutes before taking out and cool completely on a wire rack. Mix the lemon juice and confectioners' sugar in a bowl to form a glaze; drizzle this over the loaf and serve.

Chapter # 2: Flourless Chocolate Cake

Makes: 1x 10 inch round cake

Ingredients:

- 18 squares bittersweet chocolate (1 ounce each)

- ¼ teaspoon salt

- ½ cup water

- 1 cup unsalted butter

- ¾ cup white sugar

- 6 eggs

Directions:

Preheat an oven to 150 degrees Celsius and grease a 10 inch cake pan (round shape). Place a small sauce pan over medium heat and combine the salt, sugar, and water; stir the contents of the saucepan until they are completely dissolved and set the sauce pan aside. Use either a microwave oven or the top half of a boiler to melt the chocolate; pour the melted chocolate in an electric mixer. First, cut the butter into several pieces and then beat it into the chocolate, a single piece at a time. Next, beat in the sugar-water followed by the eggs, 1 at a time. Pour this batter onto the pan that was prepared earlier. Have another pan that is larger in size than the cake pan ready and put the small one in it. Fill the larger one with boiling water until half of it is filled. Bake the cake in the water at 150 degrees for about 45 minutes. The center will still look wet after the designated time but don't worry. Chill the cake, still in the pan, overnight. To unmold it, take a pan of hot water and dip the bottom of the cake in it for 10 – 15 seconds; invert the cake-pan onto a plate and serve.

Chapter # 3: Peanut Butter Cookies

Makes: 30 cookies

Prep time: 30 minutes

Cooking time: 12 minutes

Ready in: 52 minutes

Ingredients:

- 2 cups white sugar

- 2 cups peanut butter

- 4 eggs, beaten

- 2 cups chocolate chips

- 1 ½ cups chopped pecans

Directions:

Preheat an oven to 175 degrees Celsius; grease a cookie sheet. Combine the eggs, sugar, and peanut butter; mix them until they are smooth. Add in the chocolate and nuts too and spoon the dough using tablespoons onto the greased cookie sheet. Bake for 10 – 12 minutes or until the cookies turn light brown in color. Let the cookies cool for 5 – 10 minutes before removing them.

Conclusion

The Gluten-free Diet is the only effective way to counter the medical problems associated with the Celiac disease. The Celiac disease may uproot your normal routine and way of eating, but as medical treatments, like drugs, are still undergoing tests, following the Gluten-Free regimen is the only option. If you think about it the Diet is not that bad and initially there might be a few hiccups, but soon it would become a regular part of your life. It will actually provide you serenity and knowing that another bad sign of Celiac disease might not be approaching would provide you all the calm in the world.

Follow the book and live a healthy life.

References

http://nl.123rf.com/photo_19215236_gluten-voedsel-concept-op-gras-in-3d.html?term=celiac

http://nl.123rf.com/photo_30567988_.html?term=celiac

http://nl.123rf.com/photo_29466433_coeliakie.html?term=celiac%20disease

http://www.fotolia.com/id/45257208

http://www.fotolia.com/id/47136007

http://nl.123rf.com/photo_14902351_coeliakie.html?term=celiac%20disease

Author Bio

Muhammad Usman is a distinguished medical graduate of Allama Iqbal medical college (AIMC). He is a professional writer who has been in the field for more than 4 years. During this time he has produced 10,000+ articles, blogs, and eBooks on various niches related to diseases, health, fitness, nutrition, and well-being. He is a regular contributor to several journals related to medicine and surgery. He is the editor of several journals and newspapers.

Check out some of the other JD-Biz Publishing books

Gardening Series on Amazon

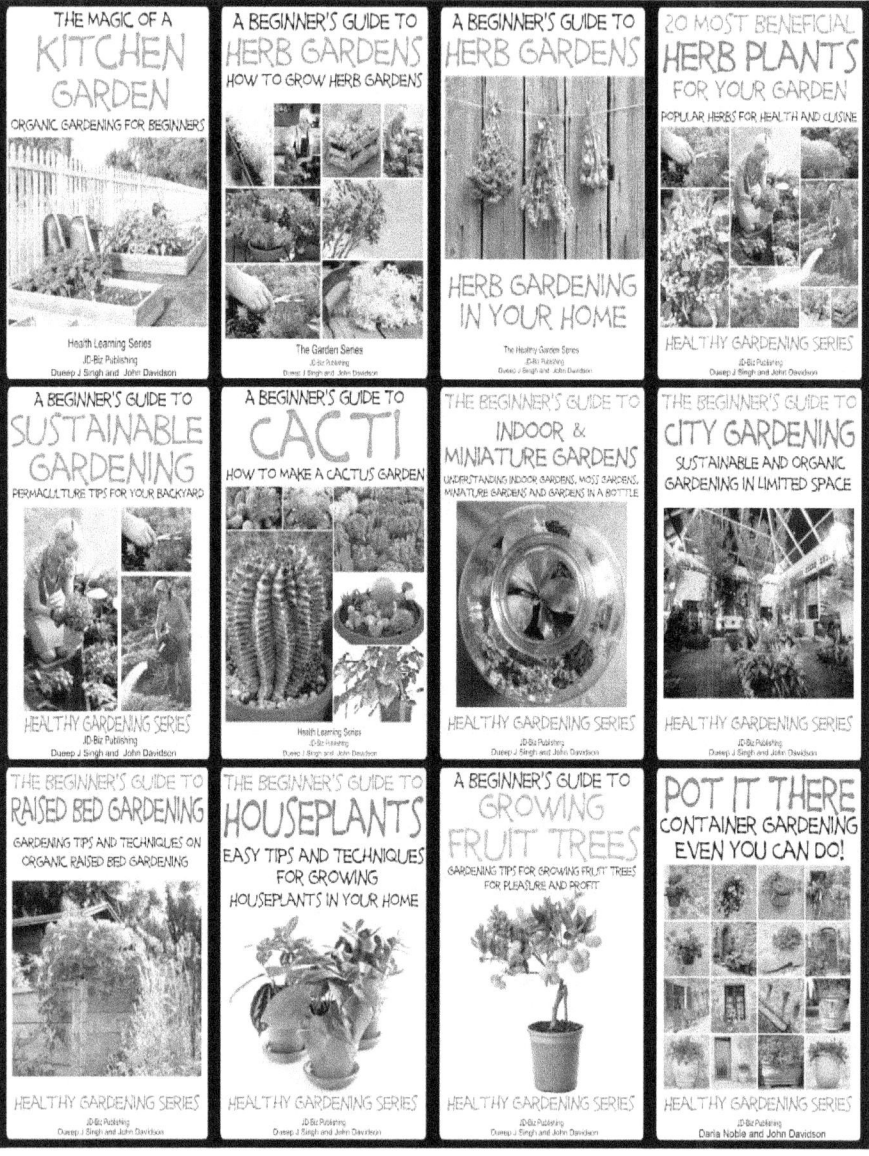

Health Learning Series

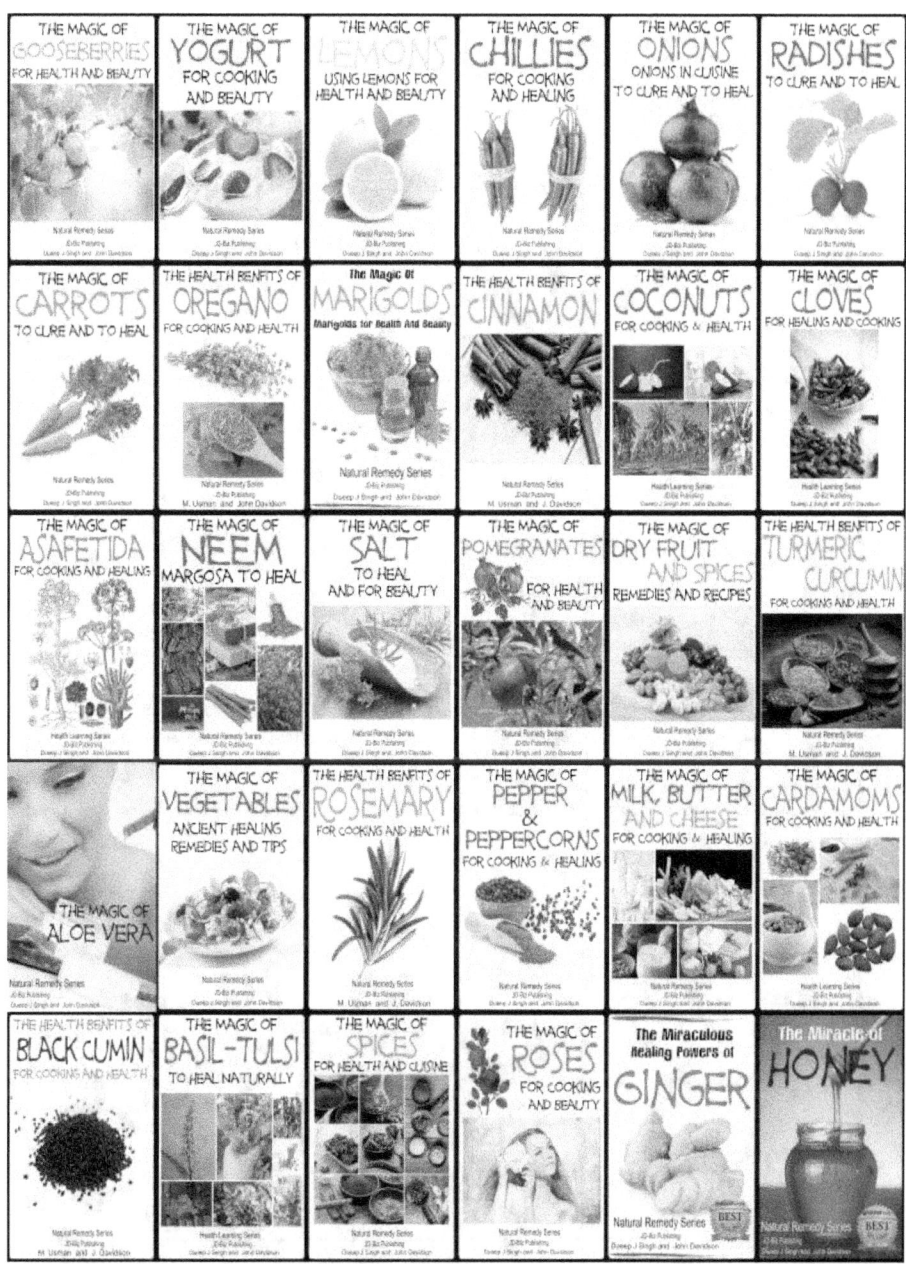

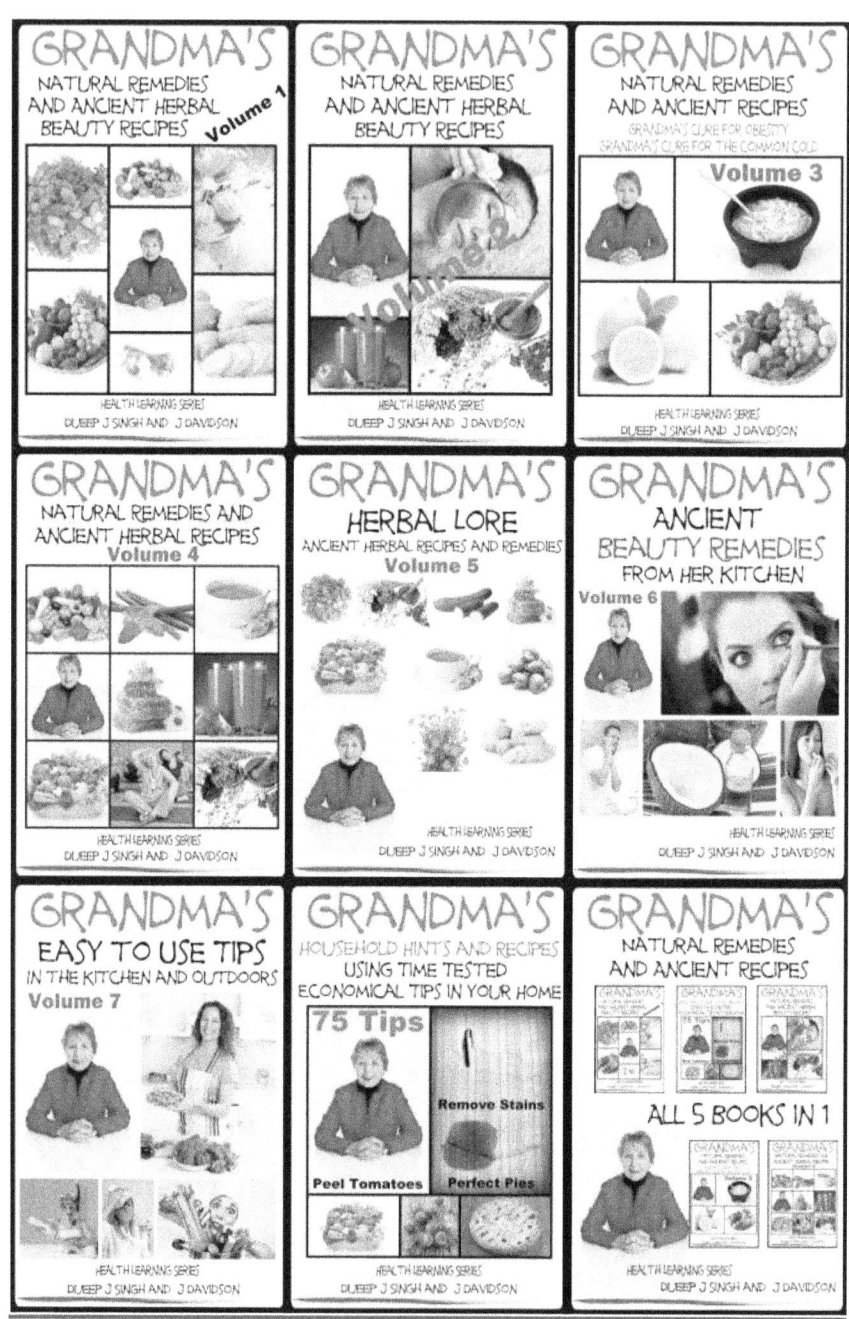

Country Life Books

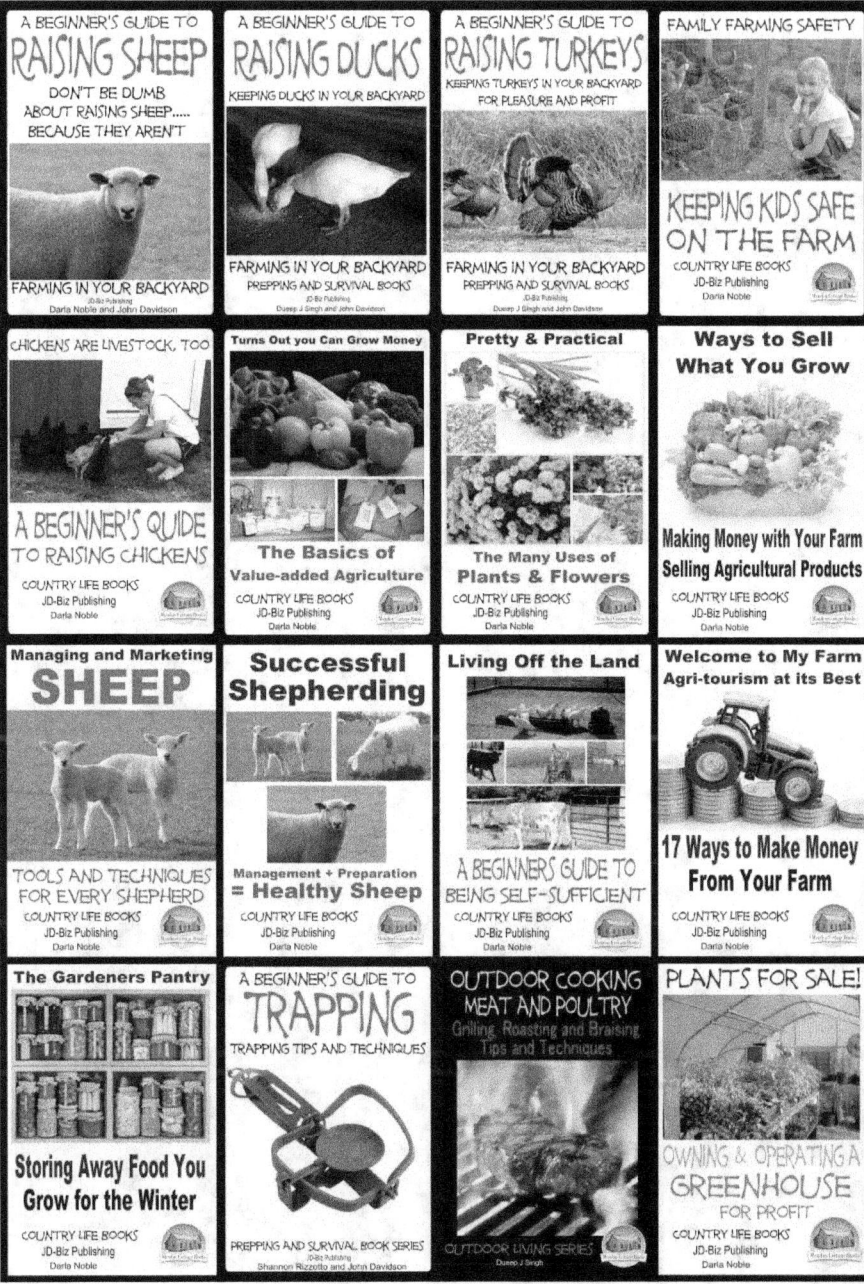

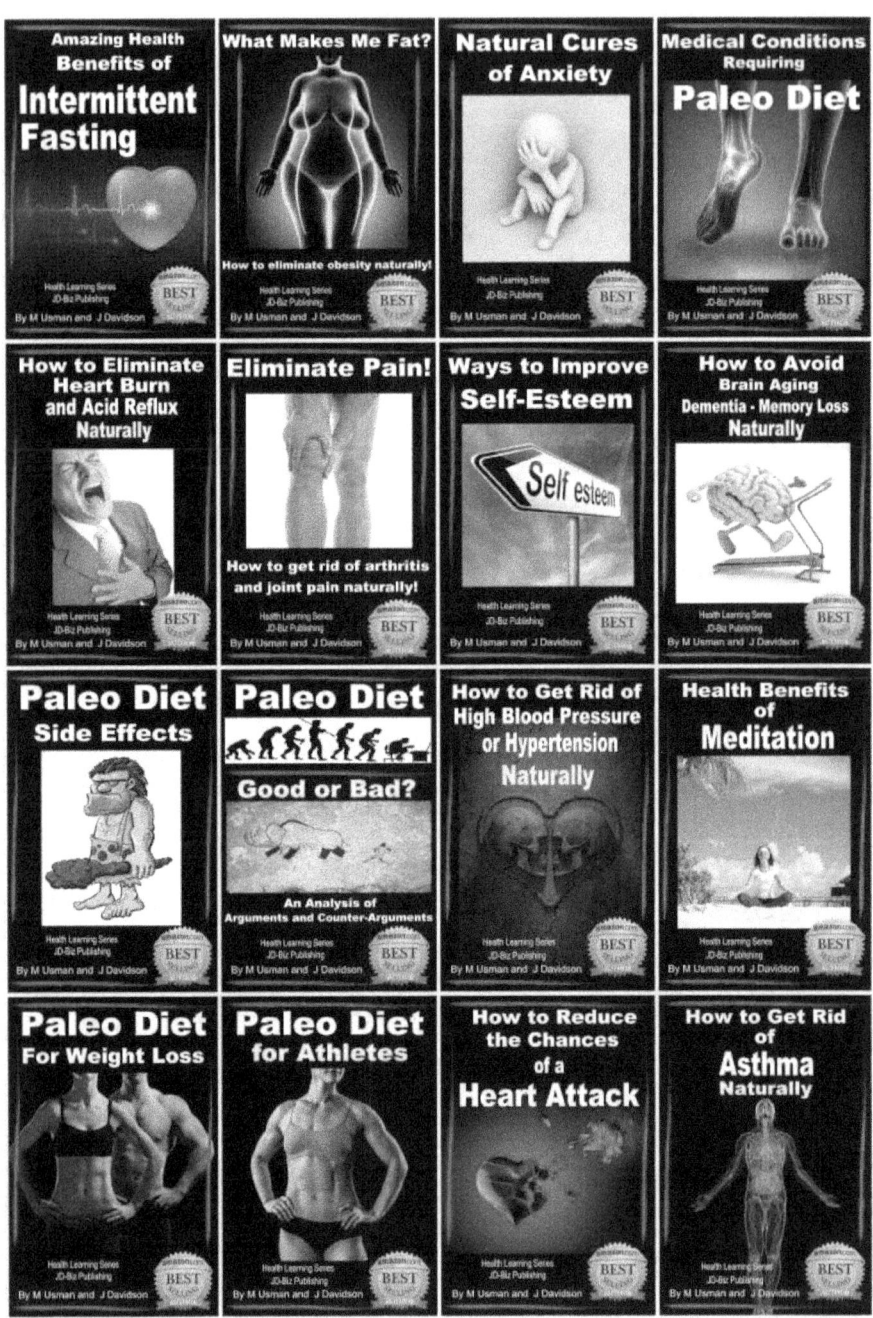

Amazing Animal Book Series

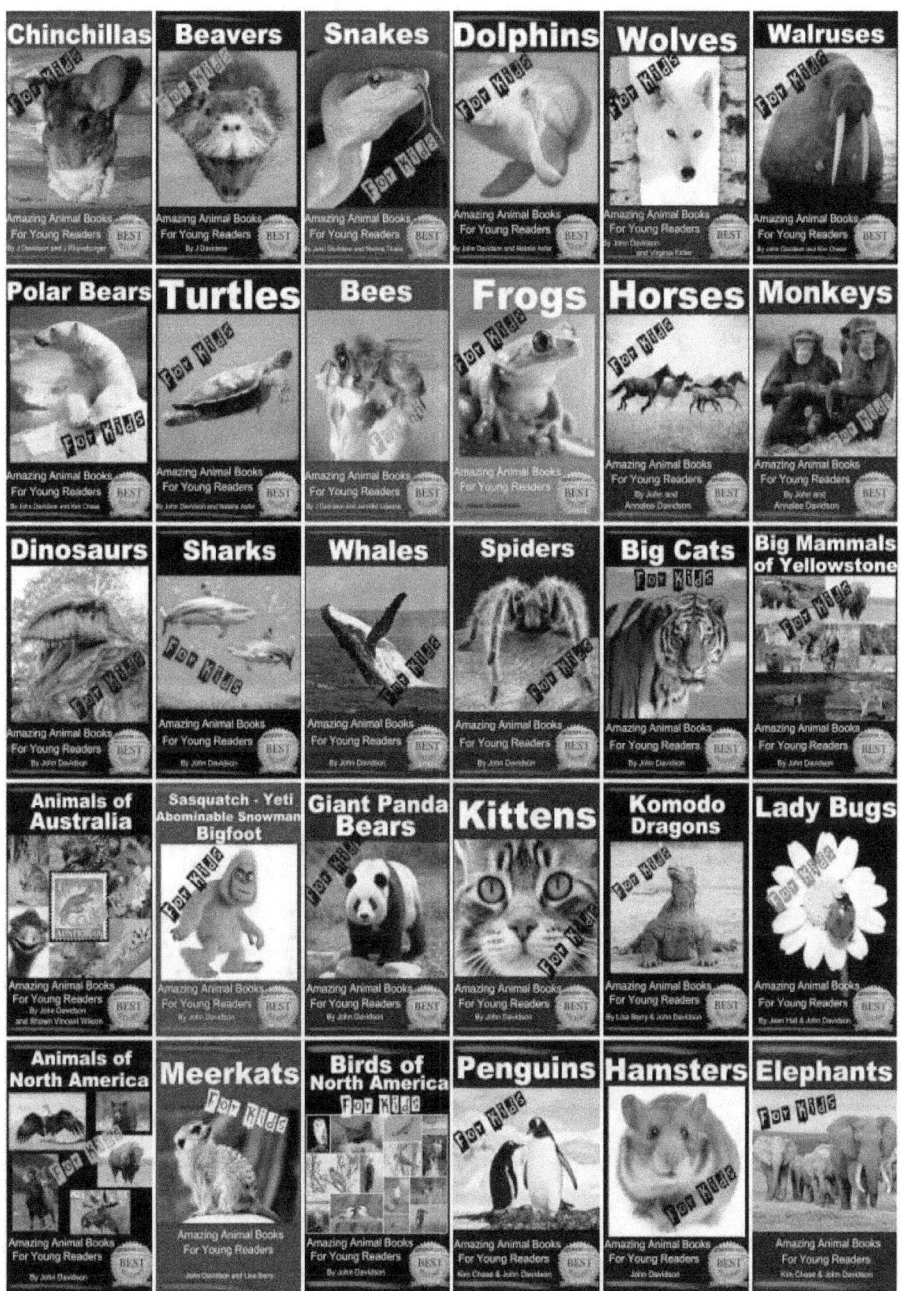

Learn To Draw Series

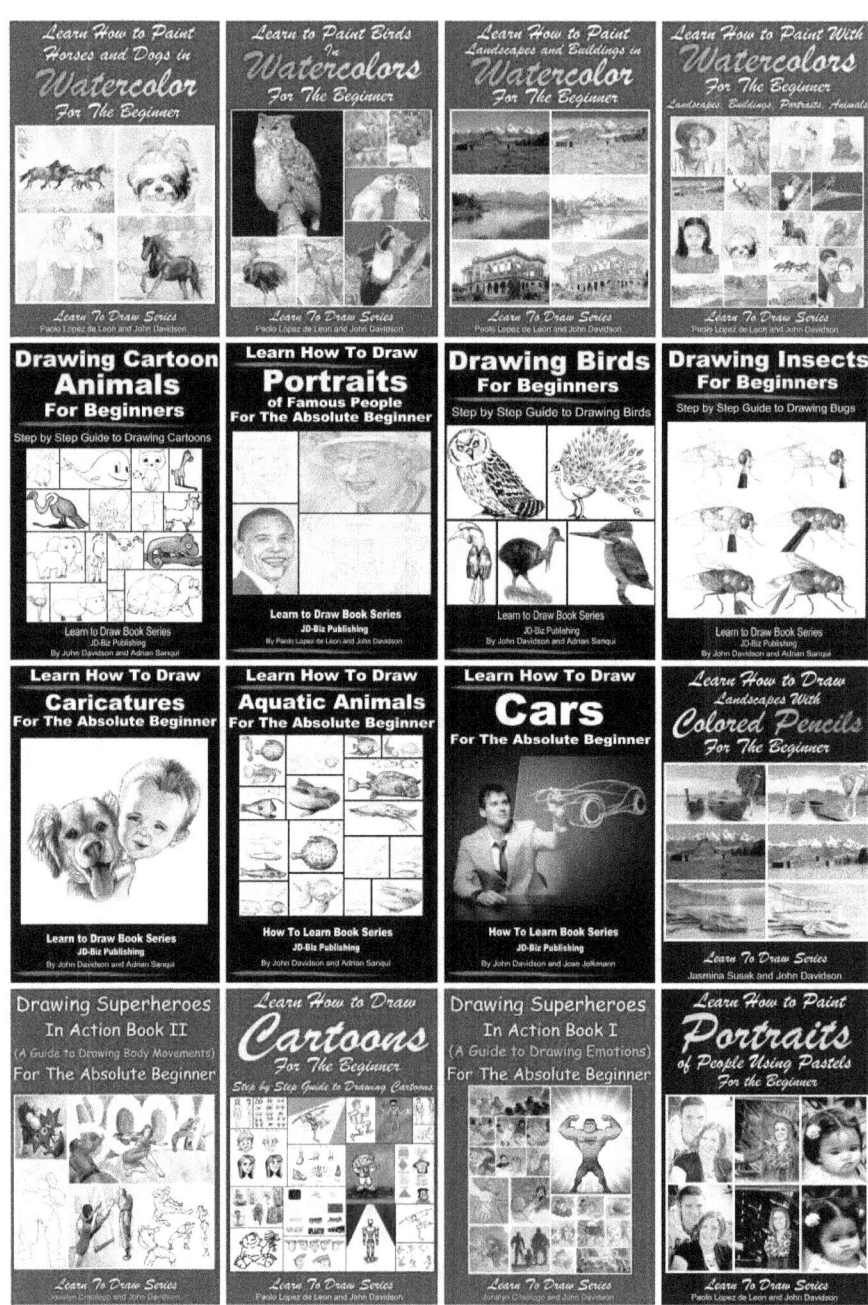

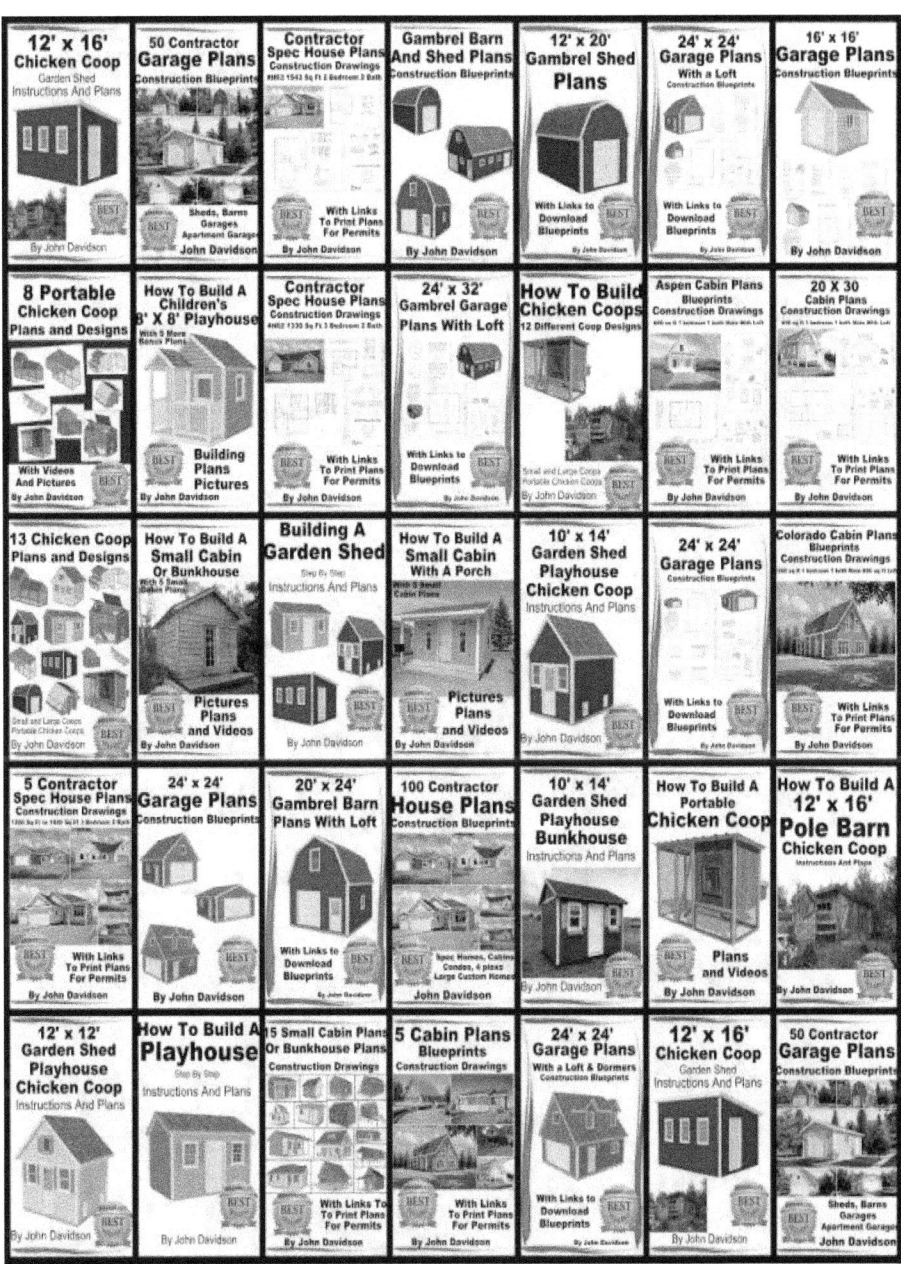

Entrepreneur Book Series

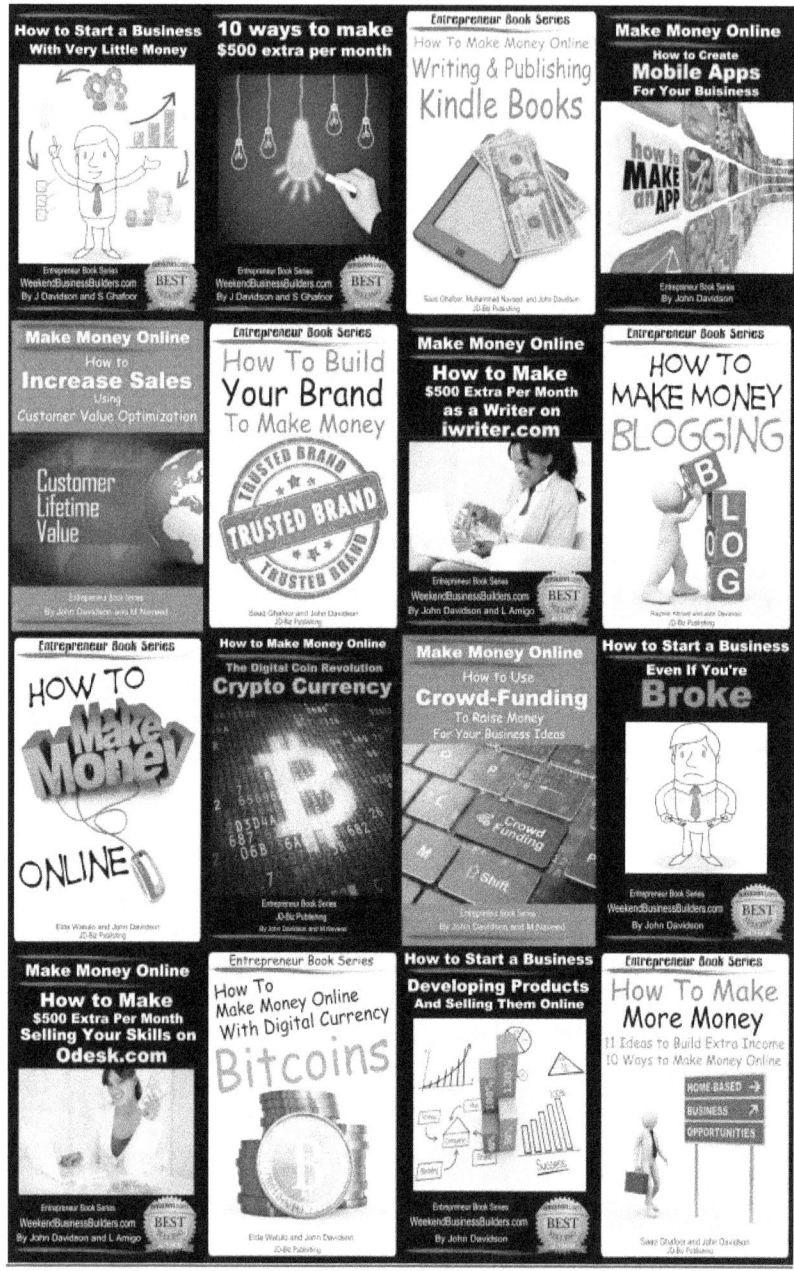

Our books are available at

1. Amazon.com

2. Barnes and Noble

3. Itunes

4. Kobo

5. Smashwords

6. Google Play Books

Publisher

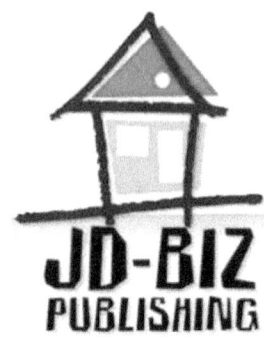

JD-Biz Corp

P O Box 374

Mendon, Utah 84325

http://www.jd-biz.com/

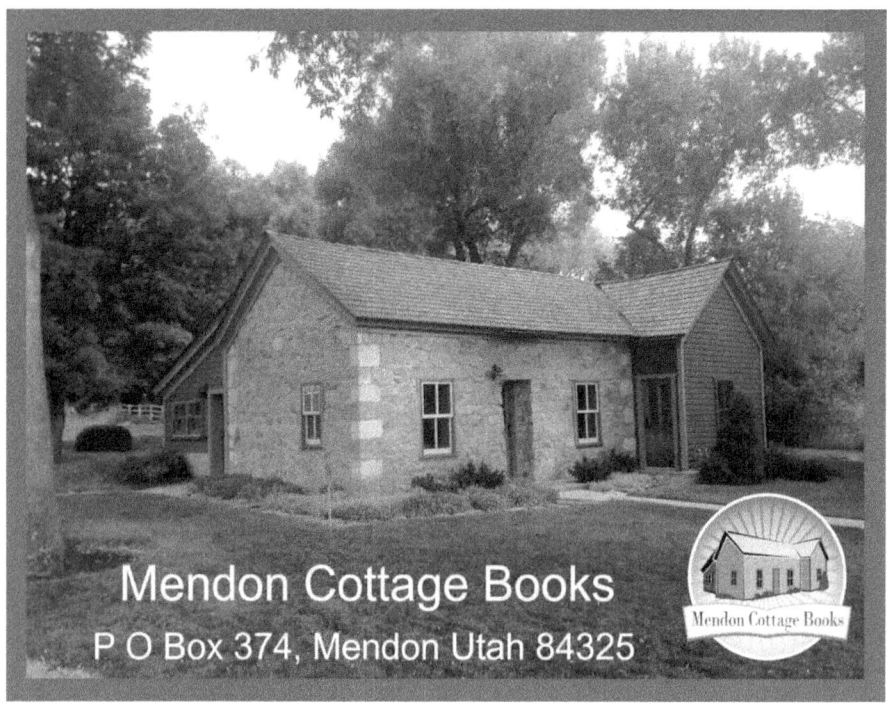

www.ingramcontent.com/pod-product-compliance
Lightning Source LLC
Chambersburg PA
CBHW071138280526
45787CB00003B/1323